Forever Young

Proven principle for a healthy lifestyle, long live and physical wellness

By : **Dr Kate D. Martins**

Table Of Content

Chapter 1
Why you should prioritise your health

Remaining solid has never been so exceptionally significant as the need to stay healthy can emphatically affect pretty much every part of our lives. Remaining fit should be possible in various ways, including eating lean and sound meats alongside a lot of foods grown from the ground. Investing a little energy every day practising can help all of us to become sound and keep away from the cutting edge scourge of corpulence.

1. Helps You Live Longer

This is one of the clearest advantages of carrying on with a sound way of life and is one of the primary justifications for why a great many people hope to practise and eat a solid eating routine. Still up in the air to benefit from their body as far as life span, there is an entire host of proof that connections remain solid with longer life. One review ventured to such an extreme as to gauge the connection between savouring liquor control, rather than smoking, practising consistently, and eating a solid eating routine can stretch out your life by as long as 14 years.

2. Feel Better About Yourself

One of the primary justifications for why remaining solid can help out to your life as you become older. One of the principal benefits is that carrying on with a sound way of life can cause you to feel more certain than any other time. Exercise can deliver chemicals to your mind that improve your temperament and give you a feeling of elation.

3. Life Insurance is Cheaper

One of the primary considerations for why remaining solid can help out to your life as you become older. One of the principal benefits is that carrying on with a sound way of life can cause you to feel more certain than any other time. Exercise can deliver chemicals to your mind that improve your temperament and give you a feeling of elation.

4. Control Your Stress

The cutting edge world we live in is without a doubt distressing, with the capacity to turn off from work being a critical issue. One of the issues confronting us is the manner by which to deal with pressure with work out. The people who carry on with a solid way of life have been demonstrated in clinical examinations to have lower levels of pressure and tension.

5. Better mental health

Great wellbeing can likewise work on your emotional well-being. At the point when you are solid, you will feel more joyful and more good, and you will be less inclined to encounter tension or gloom.

6. Reduced risk of disease

Good health assists your body with warding off sicknesses and diseases, which can assist you with remaining solid and diminish your gamble of difficult ailment.

7. Weight loss and maintenance

At the point when you are healthy, your body can consume calories all the more proficiently, which can assist you with shedding pounds or keeping up with your current weight.

8. Increase your Fertility

In the event that you are searching for a fruitful future with heaps of kids, the rec centre is the spot to go. Studies led by Harvard College specialists showed a higher sperm level among guys who exercise regularly.

9. Consider your Self-Esteem

At the point when you work-out routinely, you will as a rule find you look and feel much improved, prompting an ascent in your certainty. Higher confidence can prompt a really fulfilling life.

10. Become a Good Example

Exercising regularly and living a healthy lifestyle will rub off on those around you. When your children and grandchildren see you exercising and eating healthily, they will be more likely to follow your example.

Chapter 2
How lack of sleep can Affect your health

1. Hypertension

Getting under 5 to 6 hours of rest every night has been associated with a raised event of hypertension. Since rest helps our bodies with overseeing synthetic compounds that cause pressure, a shortfall of rest can increase the effects of weight on the body. Long stretch absence of rest has been connected with extended heartbeat, higher heartbeat and aggravation. All of this overpowers your heart.

2. Heart attack & Stroke

Rest needs cause a more critical event of destructive cardiovascular issues, for instance, coronary episodes and stroke. Trained professionals and researchers acknowledge this is because the shortfall of rest could disturb the bits of the brain which control the circulatory

system or cause bothering that makes the improvement
of a blood coagulation more likely.

3. You gain weight / Tendency of obesity

The effects of perpetual rest issues integrate fast weight
gain. A shortfall of rest is associated with higher
proportions of cortisol, a tension compound; the
resulting apprehension, stress and frustration habitually
add to significant eating and poor healthy penchants.
Another synthetic, called ghrelin, is made in the stomach
and has been connected with rest long stretch difficulty;
an overflow of ghrelin can truly make people feel more
excited.

After some time, absence of rest antagonistically impacts
the body's processing and dietary examples. Languor
regularly prompts sad longings and overindulgence,
joined by a lessening in perseverance and dynamic work.
Research has shown that people who feel unrested will
undoubtedly pick food assortments that are affluent in
carbs and sugar.

Science tells us that a decrease in work out, got together
with an extension in the total eaten notwithstanding a
development in the caloric worth of the food ingested,
ascends to weight gain. Strength is an acknowledged
best factor for sleepless individuals.

4. Diabetes

Getting the amount of 5 hours of rest around night time
is at this point adequately not. Research has shown that
absence of rest could agitate the body's procedure for
taking care of glucose which cells use for fuel and how
much insulin that the body produces. To this end it's seen
as a basic bet to figure out the improvement of type 2
diabetes.

5. Depression & Anxiety

A large number of individuals feel testy if they haven't
had a fair night's rest, at this point long stretch absence
of rest has been associated with clinical melancholy and
a more expansive loss of motivation. On the other hand,
patients with distress every now and again have
inconsistent rest plans. Rest cycles and disposition rules
are both overseen by the synthetic melatonin. Believe it
or not, lower levels of melatonin are a significant part of
the time found in people encountering horror and those
affected by a dozing issue.

Anxiety and mental episodes can similarly be a normal
reaction for people doing combating with progressing
rest need; they've been shown to have a lower ability to
bear even delicate ordinary stressors. Like despairing, at

times it might be trying to grasp which began things out:
anxiety or the rest issue.

6. Brain malfunction

After only one uncomfortable night, we have all
cultivated mental cloudiness, fatigue, trickiness and
nonappearance of focus. Right when the frontal cortex
can't rest adequately throughout a more broadened time
period, mental abilities can decrease profoundly. We
understand that adequate rest is imperative for people to
feel sharp, concentrate and learn, but it moreover
impacts our decisive abilities to reason and the ability to
deal with our sentiments and essentially choose. Fretful
people object to balance, reflexes and facilitated
developments; therefore, they are impressively more
inclined to hurt themselves. Drowsiness is a fundamental
thought in car crashes.

7. Loss of memory

Various scientists acknowledge that rest is critical for
giving the frontal cortex time to get itself straightened
out and, expressly, to commit information from the
transient memory to the really long memory. Agreeable
rest is fundamental for memory survey. Focuses on
showing improvement in mental degradation after only
one night of quiet rest.

8. Immune System Deficiency / Malfunction

Like the rest of our body, the insusceptible framework
performs best when we get sufficient rest. A drawn out
absence of rest makes a comparable response to elevated
degrees of stress; it can diminish your neutralizer
reaction and make you more powerless when you're
presented to infections, even the normal cold and flu.

9. Reduce Fertility

In addition to reducing motivation, rest issues can have a
devastating impact on anyone trying to think, including
everyone. Contraceptive chemicals are also controlled by
the same part of the brain that regulates circadian
rhythms. Getting less than seven hours of sleep every
night can result in lower levels of testosterone and the
chemicals that cause ovulation, making it much more
difficult to conceive.

10. Psychiatric Disorders

A cutoff and long stretch shortfall of rest can incite
different mental aggravations. Certain people
encountering extended seasons of absence of rest have

experienced aftereffects including disarray, doubt and mental excursions. Such incidental effects can now and again be mixed up or connected with schizophrenia.

Chapter 3
How To Improve Your sleep Habit Daily

A wonderful night's rest is similarly essentially as basic as standard activity and a solid eating schedule.

According to research, getting too little sleep can have an impact on your synthetic substances, practice execution, and frontal cortex capacity. It can also lead to weight gain and an increased risk of disease in children and adults. On the other hand, getting enough sleep can help you eat less, practise better, and be better. The quantity and quality of sleep have both decreased over the past few years. In reality, getting a good night's sleep is probably the most important thing you can do if you want to improve your health or lose weight. While many people regularly get sad rest, it is actually the most important thing.

Here are check based tips to rest better at night.

1. Increase splendid light receptiveness during the day.

Your body gets the message out around a couple of standard memories keeping clock as your circadian beat

It influences your cerebrum, body, and manufactured compounds, assisting you with remaining mindful and letting your body know whenever right now is the best, an open door to rest.

Typical daylight or mind blowing light during the day helps keep your circadian musicality solid. This further makes daytime energy, as well as evening rest quality and term

In individuals with a napping issue, daytime impressive light straightforwardness further made rest quality and term. It likewise reduced the time it took to nod off by

A comparative report in additional settled grown-ups found that 2 hours of noteworthy light straightforwardness during the day broadened how much rest by 2 hours and rest reasonability by 80%

While most evaluations impact individuals with serious rest issues, ordinary light straightforwardness will definitely assist you with night on the off chance that you experience normal rest.

Have a go at getting normal daylight openness or — on the off chance that this isn't useful — putting resources into a phoney stunning light gadget or bulbs.

Regular daylight or fake breathtaking light can moreover encourage rest quality and length, particularly in the event that you have ludicrous rest issues or a napping issue.

2. Reduce blue light transparency around evening time.

Responsiveness to light during the day is useful, yet evening light straightforwardness makes the contrary difference

Once more this is an immediate consequence of its impact on your circadian beat, fooling your cerebrum into confiding in it's still daytime. This diminishes manufactured intensifies like melatonin, which help you relax and get huge rest

Blue light — which electronic contraptions like PDAs and PCs emanate in gigantic sums — is the most staggeringly horribly frightful in such a manner.

There are two or three striking methods you can use to reduce evening blue light openness. These include:

Wear glasses that block blue light .
Download an application, for example, f.lux to obstruct blue light on your PC or PC.
Present an application that blocks blue light on your remote. These are accessible for both iPhones and Android models.
Quit looking at the television and disposition killer any astonishing lights 2 hours before making a beeline for rest.

Blue light boneheads your body into confiding in its daytime. There are different ways you can decrease blue light openness around night time.

3. Make an effort not to consume caffeine late in the day

Caffeine appreciates various advantages and is consumed by 90% of the U.S. individuals

A solitary piece can upgrade obsession, energy, and sports execution

In any case, when consumed late in the day, caffeine empowers your unmistakable system and may keep your body from commonly relaxing around evening time.

In one review, consuming caffeine as long as 6 hours before bed from an overall perspective debilitated rest quality

Caffeine can remain raised in your blood for 6-8 hours. Consequently, drinking a lot of espresso after 3-4 p.m. isn't proposed, particularly assuming you're delicate to caffeine or experience inconvenience snoozing

Assuming that you genuinely long for some espresso in the late evening or night, stay with decaffeinated espresso.

Caffeine can endlessly break down rest quality, particularly tolerating you drink monstrous totals in the late evening or night.

4. Lessen irregular or long daytime rests

While short power rests are huge, long or unconventional snoozing during the day can ominously affect your rest.

Resting in the daytime can puzzle your inside clock, recommending that you could battle to rest around evening time

Actually, in one review, people turned out to be sleepier during the day coming about to putting down for daytime rests

Another review saw that while snoozing for 30 minutes or less can upgrade daytime cerebrum capacity, longer rests can hurt flourishing and rest quality

Notwithstanding, two or three appraisals show that individuals who are known all about putting down for regular daytime rests don't encounter miserable rest quality or upset rest around evening time.

Tolerating that you put down for standard daytime rests and rest adequately, you shouldn't pressure. The impacts of resting rely on the person
Long daytime rests could forestall rest quality. Anticipating that you should encounter inconvenience resting around evening time, quit snoozing or gather your rest.

5. Endeavour to rest and wake at consistent times.

Your body's circadian perspective limits on a set circle, acclimating to dawn and dusk.

Being obvious with your rest and waking times can help significant length with resting quality

One study saw that people who had whimsical resting plans and caused an uproar in and out of town late on the completions of the week revealed unfortunate rest

Different evaluations have incorporated that whimsical rest models can change your circadian perspective and levels of melatonin, which signal your mind to rest

Assuming that you battle with rest, try to make yourself learn to wake ready to bed at equivalent times. Following a brief time frame, you may not require a watchfulness.

Try to get into a standard rest/wake cycle — particularly toward the week's end. If conceivable, try to mix regularly at a relative time dependably.

6. Take a melatonin supplements

Melatonin is a key rest substance that lets your cerebrum know whenever this second is the best an open door to relax and go to rest

Melatonin supplements are an unfathomably outstanding narcotic.

Constantly used to treat absence of rest, melatonin might be one of the most direct ways to deal with nodding off speedier

In one review, taking 2 mg of melatonin before bed moreover made rest quality and energy the following day and assisted individuals with nodding off speedier.

In another review, a significant piece of the social event nodded off speedier and had a 15% improvement in rest quality

Furthermore, no withdrawal impacts were addressed in both of the above evaluations.

Melatonin is likewise significant while making an excursion and changing according to later area, as it assists your body's circadian cadence with getting back to business as usual

In unambiguous nations, you really need an answer for melatonin. In others, melatonin is completely accessible in stores or on the web. Take around 1-5 mg 30-an hour going before bed.

Begin with a low part to evaluate your solidarity and some time later expand it logically depending upon the situation. Since melatonin could change mind science, it's suggested that you check with a clinical thought supplier before use.

You ought to besides talk with them in the event that you're considering including melatonin as a narcotic for your kid, as extended length utilisation of this redesign in kids has not been particularly examined.

Search for melatonin supplements on the web.

A melatonin supplement is a clear strategy for making rest quality and nodding off speedier. Require 1-5 mg around 30-an hour prior to going to rest.

7. Make an effort not to drink alcohol

Having alcohol around evening can negatively influence your rest and engineered compounds.

Liquor is known to cause or develop the consequences of rest apnea, wheezing, and upset rest plans.

It in this way changes evening melatonin creation, which anticipates a fundamental part in your body's circadian musicality

Another assessment found that liquor use around evening diminished the standard night levels in human improvement substance (HGH), which anticipates a segment in your circadian perspective and has different other key limits

Stay away from liquor/ alcohol before bed, as it can diminish evening melatonin creation and prompt upset rest plans.

8. Make an effort not to eat late around evening time

Eating late at night time may ominously affect both rest quality and the average appearance of HGH and melatonin

Considering everything, the quality and kind of your late-night goody could anticipate a segment too.

In one overview, a high carb dinner eaten 4 hours before bed assisted individuals with nodding off quicker

Exceptionally, one review found that a low carb diet similarly additionally made rest, showing that carbs aren't overall huge, particularly expecting that you're utilised to a low carb diet .

Consuming a huge feasting experience before bed can incite shocking rest and engineered obstruction. In any case, certain feasting encounters and snacks a few hours preceding bed could help.

9. Loosen up and clear your mind around evening time

Various individuals have a pre-rest plan that assists them with relaxing.

Relaxing strategies before bed have been displayed to moreover cultivate rest quality and are one more normal strategy used to treat a snoozing issue.

In one review, a loosening up centre around extra made rest quality individuals who were cleared out. Strategies unite zeroing in on loosening up music, looking at a book, scouring, considering, huge breathing, and depiction.

Evaluate various techniques and find what turns out to be brutal for you.

Relaxing systems before bed, including hot showers and assessment, may assist you with nodding off.

10. Block a rest time

A mysterious sickness might be the legitimization for your rest issues.

One customary issue is rest apnea, which causes conflicting and intruded on loosening up. Individuals with this issue quit breathing essentially once or twice while napping

This condition might be incredibly common. One audit guaranteed that 24% of men and 9% of ladies have rest apnea

Other normal remedially analysed issues merge rest improvement issues and circadian demeanour rest/wake issues, which are common in shift labourers.

Expecting that you've regularly battled with rest, directing your clinical advantages provider might be clever.

There are different commonplace circumstances that can cause miserable rest, including rest apnea. See a clinical advantages supplier in the event that miserable rest is a strong issue in your life.

11. Work-out regularly — but not before bed

Exercise is one of the most uncommon sciences-kept up with ways to deal with managing your rest and flourishing.

It can update all bits of rest and has been utilised to decrease side effects of absence of rest

One gather in additional settled grown-ups made sure that preparing almost isolated measure of time its expectation to nod off and permitted an additional 41 minutes of rest around evening

In individuals with over the top resting issues, practice offered a more noticeable number of advantages than most remedies. Practice decreased an entryway to nod off by 55%, complete night care by 30%, and tension by 15% while broadening altogether rest time by 18% Yet normal work-out is key for a decent night's rest, performing it too far to even consider turning around in the day could cause rest issues.

This is associated with the stimulatory impact of development, which builds sharpness and engineered substances like epinephrine and adrenaline.

In any case, two or three assessments show no hostile outcomes, so it plainly relies on the person.

Part 2 - Exercise Is Crucial

Chapter 4
Importance Of Exercise

Exercise is characterised as any development that makes your muscles work and requires your body to consume calories.

There are many kinds of active work, including swimming, running, running, strolling, and moving, to give some examples.

Being dynamic has been displayed to have numerous medical advantages, both actually and intellectually. It might try and assist you with living longer.

1. Exercise can make you feel happier

Exercise has been displayed to work on your temperament and lessening sensations of melancholy, nervousness, and stress.

It produces changes in the pieces of the mind that manage pressure and nervousness. It can likewise increment mind aversion to the chemicals serotonin and norepinephrine, which let sentiments free from despondency.

Also, exercise can expand the creation of endorphins, which are known to assist with delivering good sentiments and lessen the view of agony.

Strangely, it doesn't make any difference how extraordinary your exercise is. It appears to be that exercise can help your temperament regardless of the force of the actual work.

As a matter of fact, in a concentration of 24 ladies determined to have melancholy, exercise of any force essentially diminished sensations of gloom.

The impacts of activity on temperament are strong to the point that deciding to work out (or not) even has an effect over brief timeframes.

One survey of 19 examinations found that dynamic individuals who quit practising consistently experienced huge expansions in side effects of misery and uneasiness, even after half a month.

2. Exercise can help with weight loss

A few examinations have shown that latency is a main consideration in weight gain and heftiness .

To comprehend the impact of activity on weight decrease, it is vital to grasp the connection among exercise and energy consumption (spending).

Your body burns through energy in three ways:

- processing food
- working out
- keeping up with body capabilities, similar to your pulse and relaxing

While slimming down, a decreased calorie admission will bring down your metabolic rate, which can briefly defer weight reduction. Running against the norm, ordinary activity has been displayed to build your metabolic rate, which can consume more calories to assist you with getting in shape.

Moreover, studies have shown that consolidating oxygen consuming activity with obstruction preparation can amplify fat misfortune and bulk upkeep, which is fundamental for keeping the load off and keeping up with slender bulk.

3. Exercise is good for your muscles and bones

Exercise assumes a fundamental part in building and keeping up major areas of strength for width and bones.

Exercises like weightlifting can invigorate muscle building when matched with sufficient protein admission.

This is on the grounds that exercise assists discharge chemicals that elevate your muscles' capacity to ingest amino acids. This helps them develop and lessens their breakdown.

As individuals age, they will generally lose bulk and capability, which can prompt an expanded gamble of injury. Rehearsing standard actual work is fundamental for diminishing muscle misfortune and keeping up with strength as you age.

Practise likewise assists work with boning thickness when you're more youthful, as well as forestalling osteoporosis further down the road .

Some exploration recommends that high effect workout (like tumbling or running) or odd effect sports (like soccer and ball) may assist with advancing a higher bone

thickness than no effect sports like swimming and
cycling.

4. Exercise can increase your energy levels

Exercise can be a genuine energy supporter for some
individuals, incorporating those with different ailments.

One more established investigation discovered that a
month and a half of normal activity diminished
sensations of weakness for 36 individuals who had
detailed relentless weariness.

Also, we should not fail to remember the fabulous heart
and lung medical advantages of activity. Vigorous
activity supports the cardiovascular framework and
further develops lung wellbeing, which can altogether
assist with energy levels.

As you move more, your heart syphons more blood,
conveying more oxygen to your functioning muscles.
With ordinary activity, your heart turns out to be more
proficient and skilled at moving oxygen into your blood,
making your muscles more effective.

Over the long haul, this oxygen consuming preparation
brings about less interest on your lungs, and it requires
less energy to play out similar exercises — one reason

you're less inclined to get winded during vivacious movement.

Furthermore, practice has been displayed to increment energy levels in individuals with different circumstances, like malignant growth.

5. Exercise can reduce your risk of chronic disease

Normal activity has been displayed to further develop insulin awareness, heart wellbeing, and body organisation. It can likewise diminish pulse and cholesterol levels .

All the more explicitly, exercise can help diminish or forestall the accompanying constant ailments.

- **Type 2 diabetes**. Normal oxygen consuming activity might defer or forestall type 2 diabetes. It additionally has significant medical advantages for individuals with type 1 diabetes. Obstruction preparing for type 2 diabetes remembers enhancements for fat mass, pulse, lean weight, insulin opposition, and glycemic control.

- **Coronary illness**. Practice diminishes cardiovascular gamble factors and is likewise a restorative treatment for individuals with cardiovascular infection.

- **Many sorts of malignant growth**. Exercise can assist with diminishing the gamble of a few tumours, including bosom, colorectal, endometrial, gallbladder, kidney, lung, liver, ovarian, pancreatic, prostate, thyroid, gastric, and esophageal disease.

- **High cholesterol**. Customary moderate power actual work can build HDL (great) cholesterol while keeping up with or balancing expansions in LDL (awful) cholesterol. Research upholds the hypothesis that extreme focus high-impact movement is expected to bring down LDL levels.

- **Hypertension**: Taking part in ordinary vigorous activity can bring down resting systolic BP 5-7 mmHG among individuals with hypertension.

Conversely, an absence of standard activity — even temporarily — can prompt huge expansions in midsection fat, which might expand the gamble of type 2 diabetes and coronary illness.

That is the reason standard active work is prescribed to diminish stomach fat and reduce the gamble of fostering these circumstances.

6. Exercise can help skin health

Your skin can be impacted by how much oxidative pressure in your body.

Oxidative pressure happens when the body's cancer prevention agent protections can't totally fix the cell harm brought about by intensifiers known as free revolutionaries. This can harm the construction of the cells and adversely influence your skin.

Despite the fact that serious and thorough active work can add to oxidative harm, normal moderate activity can really build your body's creation of regular cancer prevention agents, which assist with safeguarding cells.

Similarly, exercise can invigorate blood stream and prompt skin cell transformations that can assist with postponing the presence of skin maturing.

7. Exercise can help your brain health and memory

Exercise can further develop mind capability and safeguard memory and thinking abilities.

In the first place, it builds your pulse, which advances the progression of blood and oxygen to your mind. It can likewise animate the creation of chemicals that upgrade the development of synapses.

Also, the capacity of activity to forestall persistent sickness can convert into benefits for your mind, since its capability can be impacted by these circumstances.

Ordinary active work is particularly significant in more established grown-ups since maturing — joined with oxidative pressure and aggravation — advances changes in cerebrum construction and capability.

Practice has been displayed to cause the hippocampus, a piece of the mind that is crucial for memory and learning, to fill in size, which might assist with working on mental capability in more established grown-ups.

Finally, exercise has been displayed to lessen changes in the cerebrum that can add to conditions like Alzheimer's sickness and dementia.

8. Exercise can help with relaxation and sleep quality

Regular exercise can help you unwind and rest better.

As to rest quality, the energy consumption (misfortune) that happens during exercise invigorates supportive cycles during rest.

In addition, the expansion in internal heat level that happens during exercise is remembered to further develop rest quality by assisting internal heat level with dropping during rest .

Many examinations on the impacts of exercise on rest have arrived at comparable resolutions.

One survey of six examinations found that partaking in an activity preparing program further developed self-revealed rest quality and diminished rest idleness, which is how much time it takes to nod off.

One review directed north of 4 months found that both extending and obstruction practice prompted upgrades in rest for individuals with constant sleep deprivation.

Returning to sleep subsequent to waking, rest span, and sleep quality superior after both extending and opposition work out. Uneasiness was additionally diminished in the extending bunch.

Likewise, captivating in standard activity appears to help more established grown-ups, who are frequently impacted by rest problems.

You can be adaptable or flexible with the sort of exercise you pick. Apparently either vigorous exercise alone or high-impact practice joined with obstruction preparing can both further develop rest quality.

9. Exercise can reduce pain

Albeit persistent agony can be weakening, exercise can really assist with lessening it.

Truth be told, for a long time, the suggestion for treating persistent torment was rest and idleness. In any case, ongoing examinations show that exercise eases constant agony.

Truth be told, one survey of a few examinations found that exercise can assist those with persistent torment, lessen their aggravation and work on their personal satisfaction.

A few examinations likewise demonstrate the way that exercise can assist with controlling agony related to different medical issues, including persistent low back torment, fibromyalgia, and ongoing delicate tissue shoulder jumble, to give some examples.

Moreover, active work can likewise raise torment resistance and abatement torment discernment.

10. Exercise can promote a better sex life

Participating in regular exercise can reinforce the heart, further develop blood flow, tone muscles, and upgrade adaptability, all of which can further develop your sexual coexistence.

Actual work can likewise work on sexual execution and sexual delight while expanding the recurrence of sexual action.

Strangely, one review showed that regular exercise was related with expanded sexual capability and want in 405 postmenopausal ladies.

Exercise for no less than 160 minutes out of each week north of a 6-month time frame could help fundamentally work on erectile capability in men.

Likewise, another investigation discovered that a straightforward everyday practice of a 6-minute stroll around the house assisted 41 men with decreasing their erectile brokenness side effects by 71%.

One more review exhibited that ladies with polycystic ovary condition, which can lessen sex drive, expanded their sex drive with normal obstruction preparing for a considerable length of time.

What's more, it doesn't take a lot of development to have a major effect on your wellbeing.

Assuming that you hold back nothing: 300 minutes of moderate power oxygen consuming movement every week or 75 minutes of energetic actual work spread consistently, you'll meet the Division of Wellbeing and Human Administrations' action rules for grown-ups.

Moderate power oxygen consuming movement is whatever gets your heart thumping quicker, such as strolling, cycling, or swimming. Exercises like running or partaking in a difficult wellness class count for fiery intensity.

Toss in something like 2 days of muscle-fortifying exercises including all significant muscle gatherings (legs, hips, back mid-region, chest, shoulders, and arms), and you'll surpass the proposals.

You can utilise loads, opposition groups, or your bodyweight to perform muscle-reinforcing works out. These incorporate squats, push-ups, shoulder press, chest, press, and boards.

Whether you practise a particular game or keep the rule of 150 minutes of action each week, you can definitely work on your wellbeing in numerous ways.

Chapter 5
Try These Out

Exercise is critical to great wellbeing. However, we will generally restrict ourselves to a couple of sorts of action. "Individuals do what they appreciate, or what feels the best, so a few parts of activity and wellness are overlooked. In actuality, we ought to all do heart stimulating exercise, extending, fortifying, and balance works out.

1. Aerobic exercise

Aerobic exercise , which speeds up your pulse and breathing, is significant for the overwhelming majority body capabilities. It gives your heart and lungs an exercise and increases perseverance. In the event that you're too short of breath to even consider strolling up a stairwell, that is a decent pointer that you really want more vigorous activity to assist with moulding your heart and lungs and get sufficient blood to your muscles to assist them with working proficiently.

Aerobic exercise likewise loosens up vein walls, lower pulse, consume muscle versus fat, lower glucose levels, diminish irritation, help state of mind, and raise "great" HDL cholesterol. Joined with weight reduction, it can lower "terrible" LDL cholesterol levels, as well. Over the long haul, vigorous activity decreases your gamble of coronary illness, stroke, type 2 diabetes, bosom and colon malignant growth, sadness, and falls.

Go for the gold each seven day stretch of moderate-power movement. Attempt lively strolling, swimming, running, cycling, moving, or classes like step high impact exercise.

Beginning position: Stand tall with your feet together and arms at your sides.
Movement: Twist your elbows and swing your arms as you lift your knees.
- Walk in different styles:

- Walk in a place.
- Walk four forward moving steps, and afterward four stages back.
- Walk with feet wide separated.

- Substitute walking feet wide and together (out, out, in, in).

Tips and procedures:

- Gaze directly ahead and keep your abs tight.
- Inhale serenely, and don't hold your clench hands.
- Make it more straightforward: Walk increasingly slowly and lift your knees as high.
- Make it harder: Lift your knees higher, walk quicker, and truly pump your arms

2. Strength training

As we age, we lose muscle mass. Strength training constructs it back. Normal strength training will assist you with feeling more sure and able to do day to day undertakings like conveying food, planting, and lifting heavier items around the house. Strength preparing will likewise assist you with standing up from a seat, get up off the floor, and go higher up.

Strengthening your muscles makes you more grounded, yet in addition animates bone development, brings down glucose, helps with weight control, further develops equilibrium and stance, and lessens pressure and torment in the lower back and joints.

An actual specialist can plan a strength training program that you can do a few times each week at an exercise centre, at home, or at work. It will probably incorporate body weight practices like squats, push-ups, and lurches, and practices including obstruction from a weight, a band, or a weight machine.

Keep in mind, it's critical to feel some muscle exhaustion toward the finish of the activity to ensure you are working or training the muscle bunch effectively.

Squats

Beginning position: Stand with your feet shoulder-width separated, arms at your sides.
Development: Gradually twist your hips and knees, bringing down your bum around eight inches, as though you're sitting once more into a seat. Allow your arms to swing forward to assist you with adjusting. Keep your back straight. Gradually return to the beginning position. Rehash 8-12 times.

Tips and strategies:

- Shift your weight into your heels.
- Squeeze your backside as you stand to assist you with adjusting.

Make it simpler: Sit on the edge of a seat with your feet hip-width separated and arms over your chest. Fix your muscular strength and stand up. Gradually plunk (sit) down with control.
Make it harder: Lower farther, yet not past your thighs being lined up with the floor.

3. Stretching

Stretching keeps up with adaptability. We frequently neglect that in youth when our muscles are better. Yet, gaining leads prompts a deficiency of adaptability in the muscles and ligaments. Muscles shorten and don't work as expected. That builds the gamble for muscle spasms and agony, muscle harm, strains, joint agony, and falling, and it additionally makes it intense to overcome everyday exercises, like bowing down to tie your shoes.

In like manner, stretching the muscles regularly makes them longer and more adaptable, which expands your scope of movement and lessens pain and the risk for injury.

Hold back nothing of extending consistently or possibly three or four times each week.

Warm up your muscles first, with a couple of moments of dynamic stretches — tedious movement, for example, walking set up or arm circles. That gets blood and oxygen to muscles, and makes them manageable to change.

Then, at that point, perform static stretches (standing firm on a stretch foothold for as long as 60 seconds) for the calves, the hamstrings, hip flexors, quadriceps, and the muscles of the shoulders, neck, and lower back.

Be that as it may, don't drive a stretch into the excruciating reach. That fixes the muscle and is counterproductive.

Single knee rotation

Beginning position: Lie on your back with your legs reached out on the floor.
Development: Loosen up your shoulders against the floor. Twist your left knee and put your left foot on your right thigh simply over the knee. Fix your muscular

strength, then, at that point, handle your left knee with your right hand and delicately pull it across your body toward your right side.

Hold 10 to 30 seconds.

Get back to the beginning position and rehash on the opposite side.

<u>Tips and procedures:</u>

- Stretch to the place of gentle strain, not pain.
- Attempt to keep the two shoulders level on the floor.
- To expand the stretch, glance the way inverse to your knee.

4. Balance exercises

Further developing your balance causes you to feel steadier on your feet and forestall falls. It's particularly significant as we age, when the frameworks that assist us with keeping up with balance — our vision, our internal ear, and our leg muscles and joints — will generally separate. Fortunately, preparing your balance & equilibrium can help forestall and reverse these misfortunes.

Numerous senior communities and rec centres offer equilibrium centred practice classes, like kendo (tai-chi) or yoga. It's never too soon to begin this sort of activity, regardless of whether you believe you don't have balance issues.

You can likewise go to an actual specialist, who can decide your ongoing balance abilities and recommend explicit exercise to focus on your weak spots. "That is particularly significant assuming you've had a fall or a close fall, or on the other hand on the off chance that you have a feeling of dread toward falling.

Normal balance exercise representing one foot or strolling impact point to toe, with your eyes open or shut. The actual specialist may likewise have you centre around joint adaptability, strolling on lopsided surfaces, and reinforcing leg muscles with activities, for example, squats and leg lifts. Get legitimate training prior to endeavouring any of these activities at home.

Beginning position: Stand up straight with your feet together and your hands on your hips.

Development: Lift your left knee toward the roof as high as is agreeable or until your thigh is lined up with the floor. Hold, then leisurely lower your knee to the beginning position.

Repeat the activity 3-5 times.

Then, at that point, play out the activity 3-5 times with your right leg.

Tips and methods:

- Keep your chest lifted and your shoulders down and back.
- Lift your arms out to your sides to assist you with adjusting, if necessary.
- Fix your stomach muscles all through.
- Fix the butt cheek of your standing leg for dependability.
- Inhale easily.
- Make it simpler: Clutch the rear of a seat or counter with one hand.

Make it harder: Lower your leg the entire way to the floor without contacting it. Similarly for all intents and purposes going to contact, lift your leg once more.

Part 3 - Mental Health

Chapter 6
Why you should consider your mental health

1 . Mental Health plays a crucial role in relationships

The connection between emotional wellness and relationship is one of the most convincing explanations behind its significance. Psychological instability could affect how we interface with our loved ones. Psychological illnesses much of the time bring about uninvolved forcefulness, antagonism, and the inadequacy to take part in friendly exercises. This might bring about clashes with our loved ones. Psychological sickness can possibly propel us to oust our friends and family for reasons unknown. Taking care of oneself for emotional well-being and, if essential, prescription can assist us with living an intellectually steady presence while likewise keeping up with our connections.

2. Mental Health Affects Physical Health

Psychological instability can instigate pressure and significantly affect our resistant frameworks. Thus, our bodies capacity to adapt to disease might be imperilled. A debilitated brain can prompt nervousness and misery, the two of which can make it hard to move about and remain dynamic. The psyche body association is deep rooted, which is the reason emotional wellness mindfulness is so essential.

3. Mental Health is related to Emotional Well-Being

Each day, how you feel within is similarly significant as how physically healthy you may be. Psychological wellness guidance shows the way that a negative brain can cause you to feel down, bothered, or upset. Dealing with our close to home prosperity can assist us with being more useful and powerful working and in our day to day exercises. To keep up with track of our close to home and in general prosperity, we can look for emotional well-being guidance from companions, family, and a clinician.

4. Mental Health Awareness Can Help in Curbing Suicide Rates

According to a study by the National Alliance on Mental Health (NAMI), 46% of the people who end it all have a perceived emotional wellness condition. One more review led by the US Branch of Health and Human service saw that roughly 60% of the people who ended it all had a great shape like significant discouragement, bipolar turmoil, or dysthymia. This exhibits the connection between emotional wellness and self destruction, as well as how early clinical intercession and taking care of oneself can assist with limiting the quantity of self destruction passings. It is basic to follow ideas to keep up with our emotional well-being and to know about the psychological wellness of everyone around us consistently.

5. Mental Health is linked with Crime and Victimisation

According to certain examinations, poor emotional wellness puts one at an expanded gamble of perpetrating rough wrongdoings. It likewise prompts self-exploitation and misuse. This hazard is additionally validated assuming the individual polishes off medications and liquor and is opposed to taking prescription. Much of the time, wrongdoings by intellectually ill suited people are carried out against relatives or those inside their nearby circles. Looking for tips for psychological well-being from a clinical expert and understanding the reason why

psychological well-being is significant can help in
staying away from such situations. .

6. Mental Health is connected to Productivity and Financial Stability

One of the many justifications for why it's urgent to care
for your emotional wellness is that it supports your
general efficiency and monetary security. According to
research published in the American Journal of Psychiatry
those with serious mental illnesses acquire 40% not
exactly those in great psychological wellness. As per the
World Wellbeing Association, just about 200 million
normal working days are lost every year attributable to
wretchedness alone. It is commonly realised that poor
emotional wellness causes a drop in efficiency, which
affects monetary dependability. It is important that we
do the fitting things for emotional well-being to get solid
work execution and monetary security.

7. Mental Health is linked to Societal Factors

As recently expressed, poor emotional wellness can
prompt an expansion in wrongdoing and savagery.
Offspring of grown-ups with mental issues, then again,
are bound to encounter misuse, disregard, and conduct

issues. They are probably going to grow up to be intricate individuals who battle to track down cultural acknowledgment and backing. It has likewise been noticed that individuals who are having mental hardships become socially secluded and find it challenging to keep a solid public activity. All in all, psychological wellness issues can have a critical cultural effect. Accordingly, it's basic to figure out how to keep up with incredible emotional wellness and look for clinical guidance regarding the matter.

8. Mental Health affects the Quality of Life

From the above conversation, it is clear why dealing with your emotional wellness is significant. An undesirable psyche can make us lose interest in the things we once delighted in. It can prompt promising and less promising times and overpower us to a place where we can't continue with even the most essential errands. Untreated emotional wellness is frequently related to a feeling of sadness, bitterness, uselessness, sensations of responsibility, uneasiness, dread, and an apparent loss of control. It is critical to perceive these side effects and look for tips for emotional wellness from a guaranteed proficient before it is past the point of no return.

9. Mental Health Awareness Can Help in Ending Stigma

While many individuals experience the ill effects of psychological instability, just a little rate look for treatment due to the disgrace related with it. Therefore raising emotional well-being awareness is basic. The disgrace related with psychological well-being has an effect not just on the quantity of people looking for treatment yet additionally on the assets accessible for viable treatment. For those experiencing fundamental psychological maladjustments, these might be unrealistic hardships. People can be urged to recognize their side effects, practice taking care of oneself, and look for treatment or clinical help assuming vitality by getting the message out about psychological well-being tips.

10. Mental Health Awareness enables Community Building

We can lay out better help offices for those experiencing psychological illnesses assuming we effectively crusade for why emotional wellness mindfulness is urgent. It could possibly create a more open minded and kind worldwide society, and consequently increase the possibilities of recuperation in circumstances of psychological maladjustment. Finding out about psychological well-being and showing others it will assist us with achieving a genuinely necessary change and mend the planet — each individual in turn!

Thus, when we begin focusing on our emotional wellness needs, we can make enhancements for us and for everyone around us, including:

- Working on our mind-set and mode
- Lessening our tension and anxiety
- Making an upgraded feeling of internal harmony
- Thinking all the more clearly
- Working on our connections
- Expanding our confidence

The most widely recognized emotional well-being conditions incorporate misery, nervousness, PTSD, maniacal issues, and behavioural conditions.

Chapter 7
How to Improve Your Mental Health

Sustaining your psychological health can likewise assist you with overseeing ailments that are deteriorated by pressure, similar to coronary illness, says Seponara.

Your emotional well-being can affect everything about your life, Adeeyo says, including the manners in which you view and travel through the world and your capacity to deal with the things life tosses at you.

That is the reason building propensities for better emotional well-being can have a major effect in your everyday life.

1. Get restful sleep

Rest isn't only non negotiable for physical health. It likewise assumes a fundamental part in psychological wellness.

One 2021 review remembered information from 273,695 grown-ups for the US. The specialists found that individuals who arrived at the midpoint of 6 hours of rest or less each night were around 2.5 times more likely to report continuous mental misery than the people who found the middle value of over 6 hours of rest.

The nature of your rest matters, as well: disrupted rest can add to emotional well-being side effects.

To get sufficient great rest, have a go at beginning with these propensities:

- Stay away from caffeine after 3pm
- Attempt to awaken and nod off simultaneously consistently.
- Make your room into a peaceful, unwinding, mess free space.
- Expect to keep the temperature in your room somewhere near 65°F (18.3°C).

Solid rest propensities can be more earnestly expanded all alone in the event that you have a rest problem.

In the event that you figure your resting issues might connect with a rest condition, a rest expert can offer more data about supportive proof based medicines, as mental social treatment for sleep deprivation.

Know that psychological wellness concerns can likewise prompt unfortunate rest. Thus, changes to your rest climate and evening time routine probably won't have an enduring effect. In the event that you don't see a lot of progress, interfacing with a specialist might be a useful following stage.

2. Cut back on social media

Continually consuming data about others' lives might make somebody analyse themselves and advance sensations of low self-esteem, which expands sensations of nervousness and despondency.

To invest less energy on socials, try to:

- keep your phone in a cabinet or outside your room while sleeping
- make a rundown of substitute, more significant things to supplant your typical scrolling over meetings.
- Switch off notifications or erase social applications from your phone.

3. Strengthen your relationships

People are social animals, and solid connections can impact your psychological health in different ways.

Friendship, for instance, can:

- ease sensations of forlornness
- make it simpler to get basic encouragement
- add significance to your life
- You have a lot of choices for developing positive associations and sustaining your fellowships:

- Stay in contact by checking in consistently, even with only a speedy text or entertaining meme.

- Get together for a morning walk or breakfast.
- Require a short visit during your mid-day break.

Plan fortnightly or month to month supper dates. Trying to get up to speed when you really do hang out can have an effect, as well. Research from 2018 recommends making up for lost time and messing around face to face anticipated nearer bonds far in excess of the quantity of hours members spent together.

4. Move your body on your own terms

Practice offers a scope of emotional wellness benefits, including:

- alleviating pressure
- lifting state of mind
- assisting you with nodding off quicker and rest longer
- assisting you with overseeing side effects of misery and nervousness conditions

On troublesome days, you could find it intense to do any of the abovementioned, which could aggravate you.

Movement can include something else for each individual, and it doesn't need to mean going to the rec centre — except if you really have any desire to. All things considered, make development charming for you by deciding on proactive tasks that turn out best for your body, wellbeing, and inclinations.

To get everything rolling, try different things with a scope of proactive tasks and continue to do the ones that impact you.

Charming movement could include:

- joining a running or strolling club
- taking a more slow paced supportive yoga class
- attempting situated works out
- setting up a dance party
- taking extending breaks consistently
- cultivating or accomplishing other work in your terrace
- an end of the week family climb or stroll along the ocean side

All in all, you don't need to do an overwhelming exercise to help mental health.

5. Savour nutrient-rich foods

Certain food sources can likewise influence your psychological well-being. To help worked on emotional well-being, have a go at growing your ongoing eating routine to incorporate food sources loaded with temperament supporting supplements like:

- berries
- bananas
- beans
- Whole grains
- greasy fish, similar to salmon

It can likewise serve to just ensure you fuel your body constantly — eating anything is superior to eating nothing.

Drinking a lot of water over the course of the day can likewise have benefits. At the point when you're dried out, you're denying your cerebrum and body the supplements expected to get by and work at a more ideal level.

Certain food varieties, in particular liquor, caffeine, refined carbs, and added sugars, may demolish uneasiness side effects. In this way, restricting these food varieties could assist with facilitating a portion of your side effects.

6. Know when to take it easy

On troublesome days, you could find it intense to do any of the abovementioned, which could aggravate you.

On occasions such as these, try going to humane, more open procedures, as:

- making a cleanliness pack when you can't shower --think dry cleanser and purifying body wipes.
- setting a clock to clean something for only 5 minutes
- purchasing a prepackaged feast while cooking anything feels near inconceivable

A comparative methodology you can attempt? Focus on requiring one little step consistently.

Whether it's making your bed, drinking one glass of water in the first part of the day, or writing in a diary, making this day to day vow to yourself will serve to ultimately turn into a propensity, and you will start to feel enabled.

7. Make time for rest

While what comprises "rest" may change from one individual to another, it for the most part implies offering your brain and body the chance to loosen up and reestablish.

Do you find it trying to unwind and feel rested?

Utilise the following steps:

- Lie on your back with your hands by your sides. Spread your feet separated — the distance of your hips, or a piece more extensive.
- Consider being loose, yet present. You feel quiet, yet at the same time mindful.
- Carry your regard for your actual body and afterward to your breath.
- On a breathe in, visualise a sluggish wave entering from the bottoms of your feet and going to the crown of your head.
- On the breathe out, envision a sluggish wave going from the crown of your head down to the bottoms of your feet.
- Feel your body become weighty, and remain with this casual present mindfulness for 10 to 30 minutes.

Just have a couple of moments to unwind? proposes these fast helpful practices:

- Put two hands over your heart, shut your eyes, and take a few full breaths, experiencing the glow and solace of your touch.
- Take in for 2 excludes and relax for 4 counts for 12 cycles.

8. Get some sunshine

"The sun is an extraordinary wellspring of vitamin D, and studies show it can further develop mentality and state of mind.

Your open air time doesn't need to be long, all things considered. "Five minutes of blue skies can give your care and your heart some genuine greatness."

Stuck inside day in and day out? On the off chance that you have a few minutes, I suggest:

- going for a fast stroll
- sitting in your lawn
- remaining outside taking in the fresh air

Or on the other hand, attempt these choices:

- open the window close to your work area

- propose taking a work meeting outside
- have lunch at a close by park
- Exercise outdoor

Part 4 - Your Diet

Chapter 8
Importance of a healthy diet

A healthy eating regimen normally incorporates supplement thick food sources from all of the significant nutrition classes, including lean proteins, entire grains, sound fats, and products of the soil of many tones. Smart dieting propensities likewise incorporate supplanting food varieties that contain trans fats, added salt, and sugar with additional nutritious choices.

Following a healthy eating regimen has many advantages, including major areas of strength for building, safeguarding the heart, forestalling sickness, and helping the state of mind.

1 . Heart Health

As per the Centers for Disease Control and prevention (CDC), coronary illness (heart diseases) is the main source of death for grown-ups in the US.

The American Heart Association (AHA) states that close to half of U.S. grown-ups live with some type of cardiovascular sickness.

Hypertension, or high blood pressure, is a developing concern in the U.S. The condition can prompt a coronary attack, cardiovascular breakdown, and a stroke.

It might very well be feasible to forestall up to 80% of untimely coronary illness and stroke determined to have way of life changes, like expanding active work and energising eating.

The food sources individuals eat can decrease their circulatory strain and assist with keeping their hearts solid.

The Scramble diet, or the Dietary Ways to deal with Stop Hypertension diet, incorporates a lot of hearty food varieties. The program recommendsTrusted Source:

- eating a lot of vegetables, natural products, and entire grains
- picking fat free or low fat dairy items, fish, poultry, beans, nuts, and vegetable oils
- restricting soaked and trans fat admission, like greasy meats and full-fat dairy items
- restricting beverages and food varieties that contain added sugars
- limiting sodium admission to under 2,300 milligrams each day — in a perfect world 1,500 mg everyday — and expanding utilisation of potassium, magnesium, and calcium.

High-fibre food sources are likewise significant for keeping the heart healthy.

The AHA states that dietary fibre further develops blood cholesterol and brings down the gamble of coronary illness, stroke, corpulence, and type 2 diabetes.

The clinical local area has long perceived the connection between trans fats and heart-related illnesses, like coronary illness.

Restricting specific sorts of fats can likewise further develop heart wellbeing. For example, dispensing with trans fats diminishes the degrees of low-density lipoprotein (LDL) cholesterol. This sort of cholesterol makes plaque gather inside the courses, expanding the gamble of a coronary failure and stroke.

Lessening blood pressure can likewise advance heart wellbeing. Most grown-ups may accomplish this by restricting their salt admission to something like 1,500 mg each day.

Food not manufactured adds salt to many handled and quick food varieties, and an individual who wishes to bring down their pulse ought to stay away from these items.

2 . Reduced cancer risk

An individual might eat food sources that contain cell reinforcements to assist with diminishing their gamble of creating disease by shielding their cells from harm.

The presence of free extremists in the body builds the gamble of malignant growth, yet cancer prevention agents assist with eliminating them to bring down the probability of this illness.

Numerous phytochemicals tracked down in natural products, vegetables, nuts, and vegetables go about as cell reinforcements, including beta carotene, lycopene, and vitamin A, C, and E.

As indicated by the National Cancer Institute, there are research facilities and creatures that connect specific cell reinforcements to a decreased frequency of free extreme harm because of disease. Be that as it may, human preliminaries are uncertain and specialists prompt against utilising these dietary enhancements without speaking with them first.

Food sources high in cell reinforcements include:

- berries, like blueberries and raspberries
- dull, salad greens
- pumpkin and carrots
- nuts and seeds
- Having obesity might build an individual's risk of creating malignant growth and result in more unfortunate results. Keeping a moderate weight might diminish these dangers.

In a 2014 study, specialists found that an eating regimen wealthy in organic products diminished the risk of upper gastrointestinal tract cancer.

They likewise tracked down that an eating routine wealthy in vegetables, and fibre brought down the risk of colorectal disease, while eating wealthy in fibre lessens the risk of liver cancer.

3. Better mood

Some proof recommends a cosy connection among diet and temperament.

In 2016, scientists found that eating regimens with a high glycemic load might set off expanded side effects of sorrow and exhaustion in individuals who have weight however are generally healthy.

An eating routine with a high glycemic load incorporates many refined carbs, like those tracked down in sodas, cakes, white bread, and rolls. Vegetables, entire organic products, and entire grains have a lower glycemic load.

Late exploration likewise found that diet might affect at any point blood glucose levels, insusceptible initiation, and the stomach microbiome, which might influence an individual's state of mind. The specialists likewise found that there might be a connection between additional energising eating regimens, like the Mediterranean eating routine, and better psychological wellness. While, the inverse is valid for eating less with high measures of red meat, handled, and high fat food varieties.

It is critical to take note of the fact that the scientists featured a need for additional investigation into the components that interface food and emotional wellness.

On the off chance that an individual suspects they have side effects of misery, conversing with a specialist or emotional well-being proficient may help.

3. Improved gut health

The colon is brimming with normally happening microorganisms, which play significant rolesTrusted Source in digestion and processing.

Certain types of microscopic organisms likewise produceTrusted Source nutrients K and B, which benefit the colon. They may likewise assist with battling destructive microscopic organisms and infections.

An eating regimen high in fibre may decrease irritation in the stomach. An eating regimen wealthy in stringy vegetables, natural products, vegetables, and entire grains might give a mix of prebiotics and probiotics that assist great microorganisms with flourishing in the colon.

These matured food varieties are wealthy in probioticsTrusted Source:

- yoghourt
- kimchi
- sauerkraut
- miso
- kefir

Prebiotics might assist with working on a scope of stomach related issues, including bad tempered gut condition (IBS) side effects.

4. Improved memory

A refreshing eating routine might assist with keeping up with discernment and mind wellbeing. Notwithstanding, further decisive examination is essential.

A recent report recognized supplements and food sources that safeguard against mental deterioration and dementia. The scientists viewed the following as advantageous:

- vitamin D, C, and E

- omega-3 unsaturated fats
- flavonoids and polyphenols
- fish

Among different eating regimens, the Mediterranean eating routine consolidates a considerable lot of these supplements.

5. *Weight loss*

Keeping a moderate weight can assist with lessening the risk of ongoing medical problems. An individual who has more weight or corpulence might be in danger of fostering specific circumstances, including:

- coronary illness
- type 2 diabetes
- osteoarthritis
- stroke
- hypertension
- certain psychological wellness conditions
- a few malignant growths
- Numerous fortifying food sources, including vegetables, natural products, and beans, are lower in calories than most handled food varieties.

An individual can decide their calorie prerequisites involving direction from the Dietary Rules for Americans 2020-2025.

Keeping a solid eating routine can assist an individual with remaining inside their everyday cutoff without checking their calorie consumption.

In 2018, scientists found that following an eating regimen rich in fibre and lean proteins brought about weight reduction without the requirement for checking calorie consumption.

6. Diabetes management

A healthy eating regimen might assist an individual with diabetes:

- deal with their blood glucose levels
- keep their circulatory strain and cholesterol inside target ranges
- forestall or defer intricacies of diabetes
- keep a moderate weight

Individuals with diabetes should restrict their admission of food varieties with added sugar and salt. They ought to likewise consider keeping away from broiled food varieties high in soaked and trans fats.

7. Strong bones and teeth

An eating routine with sufficient calcium and
magnesium is significant for solid bones and teeth.
Keeping the bones sound can limit the endangerment of
bone issues further down the road, like osteoporosis.

The following food sources are rich in calcium:

- dairy items
- kale
- broccoli
- canned fish with bones
- Food producers frequently sustain oats, tofu,
  and plant-based milk with calcium.

Magnesium is plentiful in numerous food sources, and
the absolute best sources include:

- verdant green vegetables
- nuts
- seeds
- entire grains

Chapter 9
How to Improve Your Diet

These down to earth tips cover the nuts and bolts of good dieting and can assist you with settling on better decisions.

The way into a sound eating regimen is to eat the perfect proportion of calories for how dynamic you are so you balance the energy you consume with the energy you use.

On the off chance that you eat or drink an excess, you'll invest on weight on the grounds that the effort you don't utilise is put away as fat. Assuming you eat and drink pretty much nothing, you'll get in shape.

You ought to likewise eat a large number of food sources to ensure you're getting a fair eating routine and your body is getting every one of the supplements it needs.

It's suggested that men have around 2,500 calories per day (10,500 kilojoules). Ladies ought to have around 2,000 calories per day (8,400 kilojoules).

Most grown-ups in the UK are eating a bigger number of calories than they need and ought to eat less calories.

1. Base your meals on higher fibre starchy carbohydrates

Boring sugars ought to make up a little more than 33% of the food you eat. They incorporate potatoes, bread, rice, pasta and cereals.

Pick higher fibre or wholegrain assortments, for example, wholewheat pasta, earthy coloured rice or potatoes with their skins on.

They contain more fibre than white or refined boring sugars and can assist you with feeling full for longer.

Attempt to incorporate something like 1 dull food with every principal feast. Certain individuals think bland food varieties are swelling, however gram for gram the starch they contain gives less than a portion of the calories of fat.

Watch out for the fats you add while you're cooking or serving these kinds of food varieties since that expands the calorie content - for instance, oil on chips, margarine on bread and smooth sauces on pasta.

2. Eat lots of fruit and veg

It's suggested that you eat something like 5 segments of different leafy foods consistently. They can be new, frozen, canned, dried or squeezed.

Getting your 5 Daily is more straightforward than it sounds. Why not hack a banana over your morning meal grain, or trade your typical early in the day nibble for a piece of new natural product?

A piece of new, canned or frozen leafy foods is 80g. A piece of dried natural product (which ought to be kept to eating times) is 30g.

A 150ml glass of natural product juice, vegetable juice or smoothie likewise considers 1 piece, yet limit the sum you have to something like 1 glass a day as these beverages are sweet and can harm your teeth.

3. *Eat more fish, including a portion of oily fish*

Fish is a decent wellspring of protein and contains numerous nutrients and minerals.

Intend to eat no less than 2 segments of fish seven days, including something like 1 piece of sleek fish.

Slick fish are high in omega-3 fats, which might assist with forestalling coronary illness.

Slick fish include:

- salmon
- trout
- herring
- sardines
- pilchards
- mackerel

Non-slick fish include:

- haddock
- plaice
- coley
- cod
- fish
- skate
- hake

You can browse new, frozen and canned, yet recall that canned and smoked fish can be high in salt.

The vast majority ought to eat more fish, yet there are suggested limits for certain kinds of fish.

4. Cut down on saturated fat and sugar

You really want some fat in your eating regimen, yet it's vital to focus on the sum and sort of fat you're eating.

There are 2 principal sorts of fat: immersed and unsaturated. An excess of soaked fat can build how much cholesterol in the blood, which expands your gamble of creating coronary illness.

By and large, men ought to have something like 30g of immersed fat a day. Overall, ladies ought to have something like 20g of immersed fat a day.

Kids younger than 11 ought to have less immersed fat than grown-ups, however a low-fat eating regimen isn't reasonable for youngsters under 5.

Soaked fat is tracked down in numerous food sources, for example,

- greasy cuts of meat
- frankfurters
- spread
- hard cheddar
- cream
- cakes

- rolls
- fat
- pies

Attempt to eat less soaked fat and pick food varieties that contain unsaturated fats all things being equal, like vegetable oils and spreads, sleek fish and avocados.

For a better decision, utilise a modest quantity of vegetable or olive oil, or decreased fat spread rather than margarine, grease or ghee.

While you're having meat, pick lean cuts and cut off any apparent fat.

A wide range of fats are high in energy, so they ought to just be eaten in modest quantities.

Sugar

Consistently polishing off food sources and savours high sugar expands your gamble of corpulence and tooth rot.

Sweet food varieties and beverages are many times high in energy (estimated in kilojoules or calories), and whenever devoured over and over again can add to

weight gain. They can likewise cause tooth rot,
particularly whenever eaten between feasts.

Free sugars are any sugars added to food varieties or
beverages, or tracked down normally in honey, syrups
and unsweetened natural product juices and smoothies.

This is the kind of sugar you ought to be eliminating, as
opposed to the sugar tracked down in leafy foods.

Many bundled food varieties and beverages contain
shockingly high measures of free sugars.

Free sugars are tracked down in numerous food varieties,
for example,

- sweet bubbly beverages
- sweet breakfast grains
- cakes
- rolls
- cakes and puddings
- desserts and chocolate
- cocktails
- Food names can help. Use them to check how
  much sugar food sources contain.

More than 22.5g of absolute sugars per 100g means the food is high in sugar, while 5g of complete sugars or less per 100g means the food is low in sugar.

5. Eat less salt: no more than 6g a day for adults

Eating an excess of salt can raise your pulse. Individuals with hypertension are bound to foster coronary illness or suffer a heart attack.

Regardless of whether you add salt to your food, you might in any case eat excessively.

Around 3/4 of the salt you eat is now in the food when you get it, like breakfast grains, soups, breads and sauces.

Use food marks to assist you with chopping down. More than 1.5g of salt per 100g means the food is high in salt.

Grown-ups and kids matured 11 and over ought to eat something like 6g of salt (about a teaspoonful) a day. More youthful kids ought to have even less.

6. Get active and be a healthy weight

As well as eating strongly, standard activity might assist with diminishing your gamble of getting serious ailments. It's likewise significant for your general wellbeing and prosperity.

Being overweight or stout can prompt medical issues, like sort 2 diabetes, certain malignant growths, coronary illness and stroke. Being underweight could likewise influence your wellbeing.

Most grown-ups need to get thinner by eating less calories.

Assuming you're attempting to get in shape, it means to eat less and be more dynamic. Eating a solid, adjusted diet can assist you with keeping a sound weight.

Check whether you're a sound load by utilising the BMI Healthy weight calculator.

Get thinner with the NHS weight reduction plan, a 12-week weight reduction guide that joins counsel on better eating and actual work.

Assuming that you're underweight, see underweight grown-ups. On the off chance that you're stressed over your weight, ask your GP or a dietitian for advice.

7. *Do not get thirsty*

You want to drink a lot of liquids to stop you getting dried out. The public authority prescribes drinking 6 to 8 glasses consistently. This is notwithstanding the liquid you get from the food you eat.

All non-cocktails count, however water, lower fat milk and lower sugar drinks, including tea and espresso, are better decisions.

Attempt to stay away from sweet delicate and bubbly beverages, as they're high in calories. They're likewise terrible for your teeth.

Indeed, even unsweetened organic product juice and smoothies are high in free sugar.

You join all our beverages from natural product juice, vegetable juice and smoothies ought not to be more than 150ml per day, which is a little glass.

Make sure to drink more liquids during warm climates or while working out.

8. Do not skip breakfast

Certain individuals skip breakfast since they think it'll assist them with getting thinner.

Be that as it may, a solid breakfast high in fibre and low in fat, sugar and salt can shape part of a decent eating routine, and can assist you with getting the supplements you want for good wellbeing.

A whole grain lower sugar grain with semi-skimmed milk and organic product cut over the top is a scrumptious and better breakfast.

Chapter 10
The secrets to Long life

<u>Part 1 : Physical Secrets -</u>

1 . Your DNA

As you age, the terminations of your chromosomes become more limited. This describes you bound to turn as debilitated. Nonetheless, way of life changes can maintain a stimulus that makes them longer. Plus, zeroing in on show diet and exercise can assist with protecting them. The fundamental concern: Sound inclinations could slow creating at the phone level.

2. Make Friends

Here is one more motivation to be thankful for your companions: They could assist you with living longer.

Various assessments show a reasonable relationship between solid social ties and a more extended life. So make an entryway to stay in contact.

3. Avoid smoking if you are

We comprehend surrendering cigarettes can expand your life, yet by how much could dumbfound you. A 50-year English review shows the way that stopping at age 30 could give you a whole 10 years. Logically killing the unfortunate behaviour pattern at age 40, 50, or 60 can add 9, 6, or 3 years to your life, exclusively.

4. Sleep

A rest is standard in various districts of the planet, and eventually there's reasonable proof that snoozing could assist you with living longer. One review showed that people who had a standard rest were 37% less figured out how to fizzle horribly from coronary illness than individuals who seldom take a few winks. Analysts figure resting could help your heart by holding pressure engineered substances down.

5. Eat well

Individuals of Okinawa, Japan, lived longer than some other social gathering on the planet. The district's standard eating routine is the clarification. It's high in green and yellow vegetables and low in calories. Moreover, some Okinawans have a tendency to eat just 80% of the food on their plate. More youthful ages have dropped the prior ways and aren't living as expanded.

6. Exercise

Tolerating essentially briefly that you're overweight, debilitating can protect against diabetes, coronary infection, and different circumstances that request a very extensive venture off your life. Waist fat is terrible for you, so base on collapsing that extra tire. Eat more fibre and work-out routinely to shave your centre.

7. Continue Moving

The proof is clear. Individuals who exercise live longer than ordinary people who don't. Standard real work chops down your likely results of getting coronary disorder, stroke, diabetes, several sorts of contamination, and awfulness. It could endeavour to assist you with exceptional intellectual sharpness into advanced age. Ten-minute showers are fine, comparable length as they amount to around 2.5 expanded lengths of moderate exercise consistently.

8. Forgiveness

Surrendering vibes of scorn appreciates amazing veritable wellbeing benefits. Consistent scorn is related with coronary affliction, stroke, less fortunate lung success, and different issues. Absolution will diminish anxiety, lower circulatory strain, and help you with breathing significantly more without any problem. The honours will regularly go up as you age.

Part 2: Spiritual Secrets

Lovely people , you can try to experience every one of the above rules the whole day, reliably anyway not live lengthily considering the way that there's one who made you , who made the Earth , the Sky and the universe.
Yet, if he helps you , you can't live as long as you expect . He is God .

God expects you to incline in the direction of you with a long life!
Licence me in any case some hoisting news: God needs to incline in the direction of you with a long life! Take a gander at a piece of the blessed works concerning this.

Because he values me, says the Lord, "I will protect him, I will defend him, for he honours my name. With long

life I will satisfy him and show him my salvation." (
Psalms 91 : 14- 16)
In the event that you haven't given your life to Christ
,this is a chance to do so . Your life is a war zone without
him , he alone can give you consistency , long life and
all the overflow you are searching for .

Say this prayer :

*" Dear mister Jesus, I understand that I am a
miscreant and a brute , and I demand Your
exonerating and kindness. I accept that you
passed on and rose again for my offences and
sins. I leave my offences and welcome You to
come into my life. I want to trust and follow
You as my Lord and Deliverer. So be it ! "*

At this point you are saved and a long life is guaranteed
for you !

1 . Live by God's promise

Declaration is life, consequently consistently he who holds His declaration near his heart will according to a veritable point of view see "life" rub on to him. In the event that you at any point have a likely opportunity to meet my folks in regulation, you can continually not work out their right age! The two of them glance somewhere near 10 years more fiery than their age, and amigos and family members who meet them are shocked concerning the way that they continue to look more youthful over an extended time. Tolerating you to ask them the mystery, they will let you know that the key is to live by God's Responsibility. Not that they don't have clinical issues to make due, yet the entire week they decide to gather their lives in regards to what the Outpouring of God needs to say for their circumstances. Right when you show love to the Assertion of God by your fundamental consistency, it will add a long time to your life.

Proverbs 3:1-2 says: "My son , adhere to my schooling, yet keep my orders in your heart, for they will defer your life for various years and bring you flourishing daily "

2. Intentionally Admit You As You

1 Peter 3:10 says "For whoever needs to value life and live all his days, let him keep his tongue from fiendishness and his lips from telling lies."

Tolerating the words emerging out of your mouth sound like: "I'm debilitated ", "my body is ending up being more defenceless", "I feel tired persistently", "I'm in the last a great time, etc - that is the thing will turn out to be genuine in your life. Subsequently, really focus on your words! Perhaps say words like: "I'm getting more youthful. My most imperative days are ahead", "yet the youthful could feel exhausted and faint, my determination is being recharged!"

3. Fasting

Regular fasting can relentlessly impact your life, both truly and fundamentally. Analysing its genuine advantages, Minister Jentezen Franklin in his book Fasting says that fasting moves back your creating cycle. Moses stayed away from a significant part of the time, including two multi day counts of calories, and the Bible says in Deuteronomy 34:7, "Moses was 120 years of age when he died and his eyes were not feeble, nor his common power diminished."

 Serve Rodgers insinuates different prosperity advantages of fasting. It cleans your body and disposes of damages. Fasting not just obstructs mixing, whenever done unequivocally, it holds amaz-ing fixing advantages to people who endure through burden or infirmity.

4. Live Decently

The bible says in Ecclesiastes 7:18, "The individual who fears God will keep away from all limits." I have constantly gone over Christians explicitly who give no thought to their dietary models. They decide to zero in on critical perspectives and disregard the genuine body (for example they have become nonsensical according to a significant viewpoint that went against being of any typical use). Quite far, you really want to live by the Soul. Something that you will do when you live by the Soul is that you will not entertain the longings of your tissue (Galatians 5:16). You will become aware of what you put in your body. Moreover remember, everything is okay at any rate not all things are significant (1 Corinthians 10:23).

The scripture says that our body is the shelter of God (1 Corinthians 6:19) thus we should respect God with our bodies. Eat nutritious food, work-out dependably, eliminate amazing rest and stay from pressure. Be driven by the Soul here as well and you will see amazing outcomes.

5. Honour Your Father & mother

We read in Ephesians 6:1-3, "In the event that a young person respects his dad and mom, it will be great with him and he will see the worth in extensive life on the earth!"

I have a lot of models where I have seen youth and sensibly developed people not experience their relegated future since they fundamentally never saw this solicitation. Your kin may not be your ideal certified models and you most likely will not have well disposed recollections of your life as a youngster growing up with them then again. At any rate, it doesn't change God's construction to respect them.